OTHER BOOKS BY

*Jerome W. Freeman*

**POETRY**

*Something at Last (1993)*
*Easing the Edges (1994)*
*Starting from Here (1996)*

**ESSAYS**

*Come and See (1995)*
*The Colors of Care (2005)*
*Bringing Kindness to Medicine (2014)*

**ANTHOLOGY, CO-AUTHOR**

*The Call to Care (1999)*

# WHAT I FINALLY KNOW

POEMS OF

DAKOTA MEMORIES & MEDICINE

Jerome W. Freeman

HEROIC PRODUCTIONS YES!

What I Finally Know:
Poems of Dakota Memories and Medicine


ISBN-13: 978-0-9987344-1-5
ISBN-13: 978-0-9987344-2-2 (hardcover)
ISBN-13: 978-0-9987344-3-9 (ebook)

Published by
Heroic Yes! Productions LLC
San Diego, CA
www.HeroicYesProductions.com

PRINTED IN THE UNITED STATES OF AMERICA

*To Mary*

In gratitude for her love and collaboration
on everything I've written

# Contents

## SECTION III:
## MUTED CACOPHONY: AN ARTIST'S DREAM



## SECTION IV:
## JUST IN TIME



## SECTION V:
## ABOVE THE CHASM

# *Forward*

The drawing on the cover ("Road to Chamberlain") and other images in this book are the work of Carl Grupp. He is a renowned artist, teacher and wisdom seeker. I treasure his friendship and talents.

The "Road to Chamberlain" can be a metaphor for what we hope for and believe. Poetry and stories about medicine can evoke images of struggle and mortality, but also visions of kindness, meaning and survival. The Dakota prairie conjures similar themes.

SECTION I:

# The Road to Chamberlain

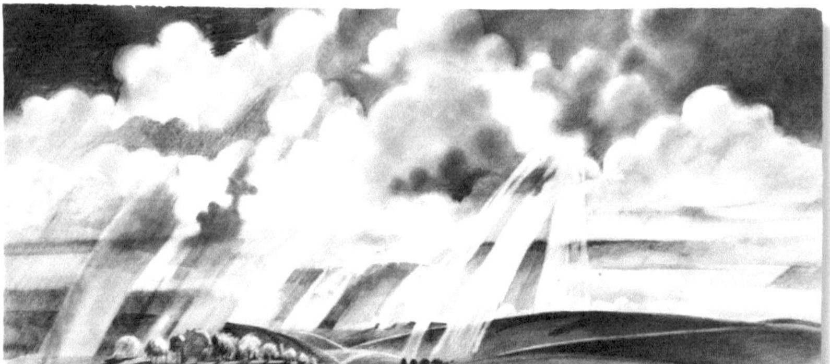

# THE ROAD TO CHAMBERLAIN

At the crest of the hill, the Missouri is a grey
ribbon, calm and confident in late afternoon.
The railway trestle parallels the new bridge,
companions under bulbous clouds and javelins
of setting sunlight. The river bluff reigns as
both destination and point of departure,
an alpha and omega vantage.

Lewis and Clark, of course, had different
perspectives from their flatboats. Wisdom
accumulated slowly as they scanned
the shoreline for omens and game.
Decisions had irrevocable consequences.
Uncertainty was everywhere.

Distracted by thoughts of other rivers,
the Rubicon and Styx, I cross the long
bridge and ascend the opposing hillside.
Possibility and stern fate still merge
together, as in the past. Life is thrilling
and fragile. The summit of the next hill
or the one beyond will herald another
vista, another river. There will be
a beginning or an end.

## INQUIRY

Everywhere in the hospital
I see myself in others' faces.
The eyes mostly give truth
away.

That stoop-shouldered man,
looking lost in front of room
306, could be me trying to
understand

how life can go on after
a thirty-year old spouse
learns a mere lump has
become cancer.

Chance casually governs
the corridors of illness.
Much is in shadow.
Everything is personal.

# ORDINARY PROCRASTINATIONS

Through the windowpane
I gaze at a night light of full
moon, unblinking in its solemn
witness to yesterday's good
intentions and missteps.

The solitary perspective is
silent, aloof to my appeals
and explanations.

I am undone or just beginning
as dawn creeps up behind
to reveal second chances.
Much is poised to happen
or not.

# THE TROJANS

It's a hard thing to suffer a war
for a woman we neither know
nor love. We were proud when
Paris bested the dirty Greeks
with her abduction, but that was
before this siege and paltry rations.

Our gods and old Priam tell us
the portents are promising.
But we are fatigued, yearning
to leave these walls and walk
along the beach alone.

Yesterday Helen passed by
the rampart looking bored and
beautiful in the morning sun.
Crazy Cassandra followed
apace calling out jealousy
and doom. All welcomed
the diversion.

Now we hear the enemy's
strange calls, amid pounding
clamor on the plains. This
latest project will surely fail
like their earlier machinations.
Maybe then the horde will return
vanquished to their distant home
and deserted women, if they will
take them back again.

## MAKING IT SO

*At the dedication of the medical school's Wegner Library*

These grand walls circle our enthusiasm
as we gather to affirm our belief in where
we're going. Always we are learning to
see the world in new ways. Sometimes
truth is where we seek it, as we yearn
for better ways to care.

Hard lessons teach us that much can go
wrong. Intentions are fragile. Success,
when achieved, is a shared glory.
Failure, when it seeps into our projects
insists on more solitary torments. Many
days test the limits of our contentment.

But today collegial tiers of windows focus
confidence and light upon our assembly,
as we celebrate unseen connections
to everywhere. We breathe the rarefied
air of the possible, before dispersing
to the unsettled lives of those we serve.

# THE BOLO

The bolo tie is understated
in a brash sort of way, as if
saying too much and too
little at the same time.

Each cervical signature
encircles the bearer with
affability that feigns humility,
while pleading for comment.

For human endeavor and
neckwear, failure hovers
perilously close to stunning
success.  Choice matters.

# PARTING DECLARATION

The grove protects a weary crease
of April snow as meadow grass creeps
forward like a vanguard of Lilliputians
surrounding a slumbering giant doomed
to melt soon from memory.

Elsewhere around the world time-weary
patriarchs pace the periphery of former
influence, cursing frailty and callow forces
marshaled against them.

Life is grand and cyclical and somber.
Seasons soldier on, failing to note
successive departures

SECTION II:

# Words Spew Forth in Volcanic Wonder

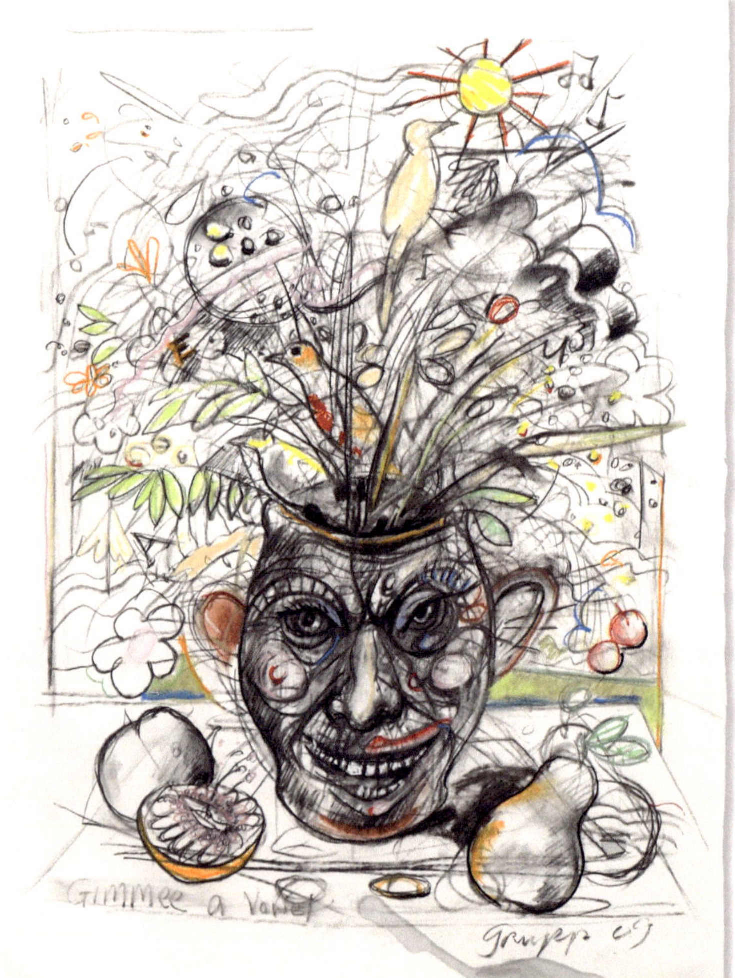

Gimmee a

# WORDS SPEW FORTH IN VOLCANIC WONDER

What I mean to report
are things I believe at night
when facades crumble.
Phrases appear amid
the debris.

Words can mean anything
depending on how they're
strung together. At best,
metaphor is a half truth.
Ardor falters.

To say I love you
presumes our meanings
converge. They may,
just prior to an eruption
of disharmony.

Retorts grow mean.
So we realign our lives
to grasp mere vowels
and consonants as props
for saying it better.

## SOCIAL GALAXY

At the reception
we stand nervously
near one another
reciting pleasantries
and plotting gracious
excuses to move on
to brighter stars.

## MENTORING A MEDICAL STUDENT

Before you were listening
you studied the history sheet
more than the patient, careful
to check off items about each
organ system.

Before you were listening
you were sure of an answer
before the question was even
asked. Your confidence
drowned whispers of sorrow.

Before you were listening
your world was preoccupied
with competing views and
voices. You sometimes mistook
an appeal for idle conversation.

Before you were listening
you were deaf to essentials,
callow but not calloused.
What you didn't hear,
made a difference.

## THE POETRY CRITIC

She lives in a world of canny
craftsmanship and subdued spirit.
Meaning dangles precariously
and hubris hovers about.

She either likes a poem upon
first cursory review or summarily
dismisses it with arbitrary and
comfortable assurance.

Sometimes she grasps a gem,
a wordsmith's triumph, and clasps
it to her chest, making it her own.

# FAIR APPRAISAL

What's fair about a bad back or
breast cancer at age 38 or
a heart that sputters and rues
the loss of regular rhythm?

Some things just don't work out.
Even the optimist can see that.
Odds seem precariously stacked.

The truth about the truth waylays
dreams.  Remorse settles in and
accounting for losses is completed
by dawn, just before morning coffee.

## ON LEARNING THE DIAGNOSIS

From here to the corner the world is familiar.
Security is etched onto storefronts.
An occasional canopy juts out just where
it's needed to protect from weather.
Unexpected sidewalk irregularities lie
in sunlight and are easily avoided.

At the end of the block, you turn onto
an uncertain street, locked in shadows.
Your diagnosis is not death itself, but feels like it.
Eyes that formerly scanned a neighborhood
now struggle to peer inward, as if your bones
suspend a timetable for coming decline like

Union Station posts schedules for departing
trains.  People passing by seem immune
from apprehensions about health.
Their everyday thoughts are not roiling
like yours.  City facades continue to focus
their attention.

# A LEGAL QUESTION FOR MEAD BAILEY

A barbed wire fence ran across
the old right-of-way road when
we bought the adjoining land in 1975.
A farm-to-market road, our neighbor,
Mead said.  Probably the bridge washed
out in the 40s when the creek changed
course.  Mead, who had answers for most
things, didn't know for sure.

We adopted the roadway as our own
over the years, a private path to the creek.
This week, on three consecutive days,
unsigned notes appeared, stuck onto
rusted barbed wire.  Remove this fence,
commanded the first.  Then, you will
be responsible if someone gets hurt here.
And finally, this is public property.

Mead, wise and lawyerly, pondered
such remonstrance with great interest.
Often his declarations were terse.
Asked if such anonymous accusations
were valid, he authoritatively opined,
maybe and maybe not.

## TRIBUTE, 1998

*for Jason*

Tonight, amid leftovers and wine,
I finally read your summer collection,
expecting I could anticipate your style
and vision, only to be overturned
by your art, and all the time wondering
how you know such things and how
you pull from your soul phrases so
searing that deceit and perdition quake
at the prospect of being branded by
your images as they rile the mundane
to demonstrate it's not our ordinary
failures that require camouflage but all
lost opportunities to act with kindness.

SECTION III:

# Muted Cacophony: An Artist's Dream

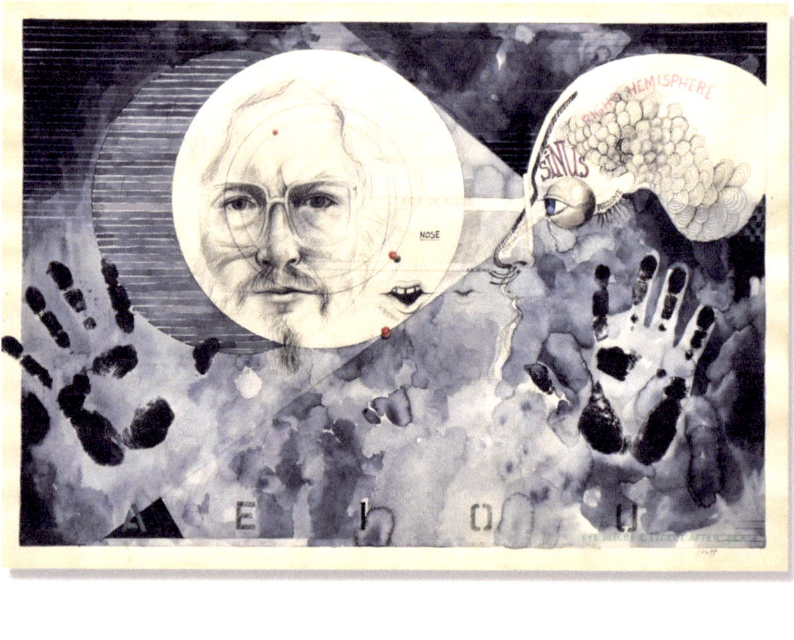
NOSE
SINUS
HEMISPHERE
A E I O U

# MUTED CACOPHONY: AN ARTIST'S DREAM

Look first at the eyes, the portal
to what lies behind appearances.
Who are you (one might innocently
inquire) and what are your intentions?
Your lips move like ripples, almost
imperceptible against the opaque
backdrop of your life. Spell it out
if you dare. Vowels of imagination
align themselves in silent cadence
on your horizon. Watch carefully.

Details of anatomy are better
visualized than discussed.
All meaning can be given dimensions.
Extended hands gesture welcome
or stern warning against intrusion.
You scowl at the notion that sound can't be visual.
There's more here than meets the ear.
The clamor of competing voices wanes.
To see is to know.

# AT THE SYMPHONY

Pausing after the first movement,
the conductor mops his brow
and nods to the musicians,
while the audience enjoys
a cacophony of throat clearing
and program rustling in preparation
for sitting soundlessly again.

## ANOTHER COLLABORATION

*for Carl Grupp*

You can go first, I say
thinking it's easier to wrap
words around a painting than
the other way. You could do
a self portrait like the old days.
He likes the suggestion and replies
I can't get enough of myself.
But as he paints and I worry
over his shoulder some other
figure appears to perch on
the edge of life. If you want
profound it costs more, he says
as he measures life in rapid strokes,
recalling a Mexican mask once hung
on the wall to a wife's dismay.
Her illusions weren't mine.

# HICCUPS

Abruptly they appear again
in gusts that ruffle leaves
and strain the roots of the body.

Each strong rush seems to climb
on the back of its predecessor
to better survey the chaos.

The green and calm of routine
tumbles before the storm.
A fearful query stirs somewhere

beneath the surface. What if this
tumult does't finally blow over
this time as it always has before?

# PERSPECTIVE

I hate people who think
they know it all and act
better than me, holding
their noses tilted skyward
as if to better sniff the air
about me, while I'm thinking
"Hey, I need to breathe too
you pompous pundit."

But of course I don't actually
speak.  Instead, I lean back
and smile at their presumption
of having every answer, while
knowing all along that I do.

# AT THE MS CLINIC

Signs are protean, like syphilis, like fear.
Numbness creeps into consciousness.
A careless stumble is a caution

as two roads, then four, then more diverge.
Destination is veiled, receding before
each hopeful advance.  Illusions chafe.

The broad sweep of life is constrained
by ill-timed exacerbations.  Threat of
inexorable erosion lingers fiercely.

## STILL

She lies upon the rumpled bed,
locating herself in the morning.
The night has issued a reprieve.
She remains as she was.

If the renegade cells have
advanced their cause while
she slept, it is not yet evident.

The early breeze is sweetness
in sunshine. Health is more
fragile than hope, than love.

SECTION IV:

# Just in Time

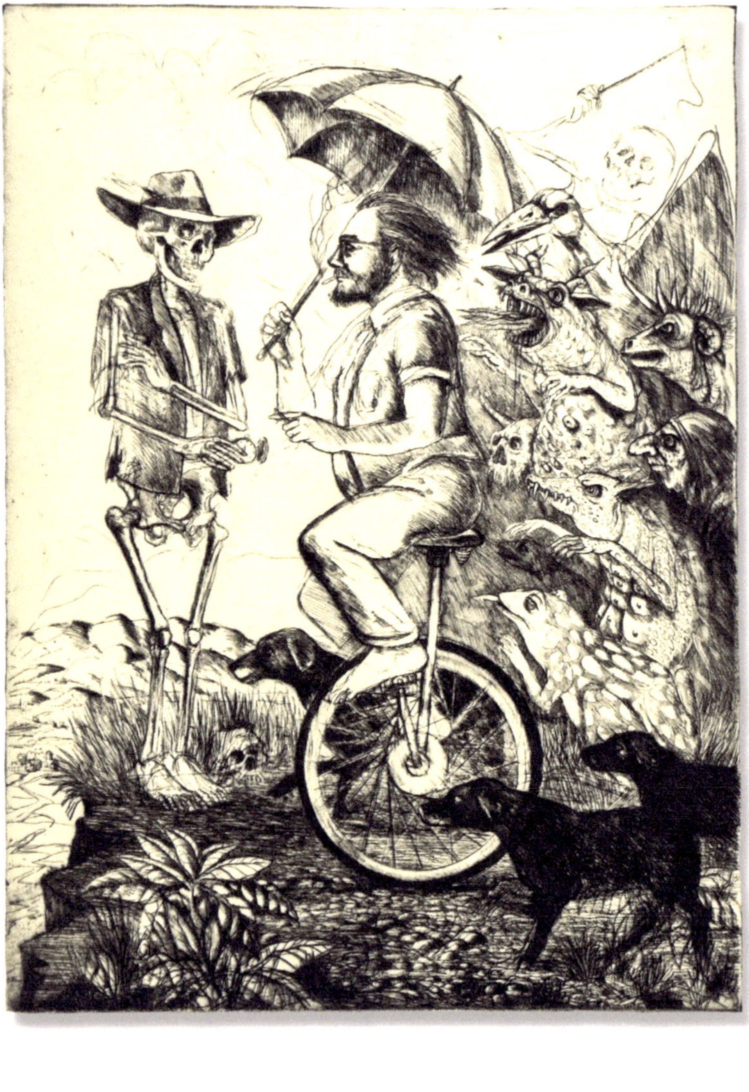

## JUST IN TIME

Time is relative when
you think you've got
all you need.

It's the limits that will
get you in the end,
roil a sour stomach,
keep you awake at night.

When the perimeter is
in sight, a stride or two
away, you'll falter and
glance backward.

Destiny foretells regrets,
the coming of grief,
deferred reunion.

## MAKING ASSUMPTIONS

For the first ten minutes I am patient,
glancing at the menu and toward
the languid street, still fatigued
from rush-hour traffic.

Then a prickle of concern begins.
Has she forgotten or deferred
to a more pressing commitment?
The couples at the adjoining tables

casually consider my dilemma
and choice of wine while feigning
disinterest. Properly chic, they refrain
from audible conjectures.

Finally I depart in the ordinary way
with mumbled excuses and glances at
my watch. At the doorway, I remember
to turn back and settle my account.

# OFF WARRANTY

If you'd just come in sooner, we
could have helped. Commerce and
custom accept that all things wear out.
You should have adhered to stipulations.

A variance of the heart may count,
or not. The body insists on its own
rules. Rhythms of obsolescence prevail.

If the pendulum of regularity is jostled,
the secure arc wobbles on new physics.
Design falters. The EKG keeps time
to the beat, oblivious of consequences.

## THE WAY WE LIVE

Cancer has made me his confessor.
As I sit by the bedside, he numbers
indiscretions, data for diagnosis.

The push and pull of an ordinary life
is revealed. What was cherished
seems squandered, as he bargains

for a second chance. Things could
surely be different next time, each
promise kept, priorities reordered.

He yearns for a permanence of things.
The pale and predictable are enough,
certain grace for another morning.

# THE OFFICE PARTY DURING CHRISTMAS SEASON

Together we linger in the doorway
to watch coworkers weave a tapestry
of lives. Some call greetings across
the room, while others nod or touch
a forearm in gentle emphasis.

A moratorium on protocols and
deadlines is celebrated, while unity
of purpose seems possible. At evening's
end, couples descend the stairs arm in arm
to encounter who they may become.

## ON DEPRESSION

You could see tragedy coming
from a distance slowly, like
a wagon train inching in and out
of view over undulating prairie.

Warning calls were muted
by your remove and distraction.
By the time depression settled in,
it seemed too late to act or care.

Important things were lost,
as when the perfect phrase
comes to the writer just before
sleep and is forgotten by dawn.

In the ample night you awaken
still to strains of uncertainty.
Your compass is awry and much
can go wrong. If something matters

now, it's the practical. Where
to draw the line. How to learn
the nuances of things. Whether
to start over.

## TUNNEL VISION

There's much we don't see,
like innocence beneath a wry
retort or pasque flowers
hidden under prairie grasses.

A perfunctory glance may miss
earnest plans for starting over
or an owl atop a fence post.

Perspective can be distorted by
prospects of our own failure
and threat of malign influences.

We teeter precariously, only
to refocus on ordinary wonders
like a blue heron and scalloped hills
stretching across the horizon.

# THIS TOO CAN HAPPEN

We arise each morning ordinary
and tousled by sleep.  We are
equal more or less in our groans
and ablutions.  What distinguishes
is what happens later, during chance
encounters, with a business
handshake, after a goodbye kiss.

A matter-of-fact day wobbles
forward, not planning on surprise.
Then someone steps softly around
obstacles to make things right by
ferociously summoning change.
Fate is fashioned by mundane
and marvelous acts.

## DEMENTIA UNDONE

Maybe he'll snap out of it
some say, implying that he
might abruptly stand and
dust off his clothes and look
about for a morning paper.
Then, enroute to the coffee shop,
he'll pause to smell lilacs again,
marveling at purple on green
on springtime display.

His grandson, bearing patient
vigil for this resurrection, still
expects to get his hair playfully
mussed again if he waits long
enough.

SECTION V:

# Above the Chasm

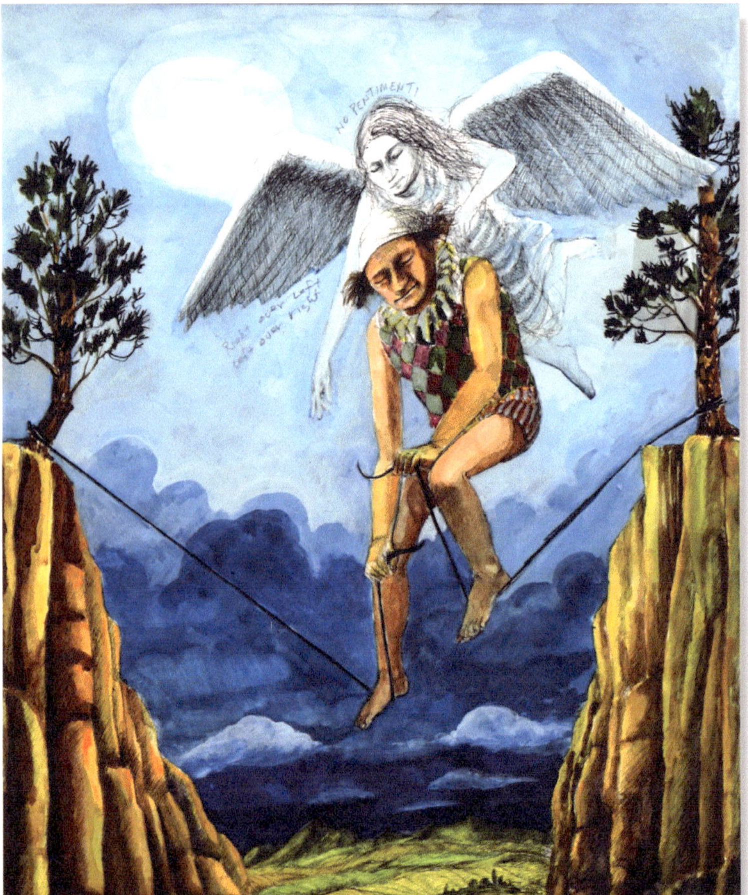
NO PENTIMENTI
Right over Left
Left over Right

## ABOVE THE CHASM

When feeling most fragile, you're often
alone, confronting personal demons
or the burdens of a fickle world.
There is little difference.

Summon your wits.  Take any help offered.
Don't make a Gordian knot when a square
knot is needed.  Remember they're not
interchangeable.

Abandon all forecasts of the future.
Predictions are wobbly refuge,
bandied about to thwart decisive
action.  Avoid delays.

And don't forget to look down.
The view will focus attention if you're
headed for a fall.  Consequences may be
worse than you fear.

Expect surprises.  Motivations are
oblique and subject to change.
Gentle hands may extend to cushion
your descent.

## UNCOMMON ELEGY

Being used to sadness probably
prepared him for those later years
of having money but not much
to spend it on. Alone, he had
few places to visit or people to see,
including the children who lived
apart in miles and spirit.

It became easier to talk about
family than to be together,
to suffer noble isolation in schemes
and visions that remained illusory.
He was Sisyphus, tumbling down
from a height each time he sought
the final handhold.

He was different after the war
his sisters said, something changed.
Perhaps the will to laugh at himself
was drowned in the seriousness
of getting by. He sensed betrayal
as presumed destiny blinked
and looked away.

Always when I pass a train hurdling
in the opposite direction, I think
of his explanations of relativity
to vaguely attentive children in
the back seat. We, who grew up
in our own ways relative to
his wishes and distractions,

mostly turned out like he'd planned.
Even after rejecting his advice, we
often returned to it. While offering
foresight for his children, he lacked
vision for himself. As independence
slipped away he wrote ferociously
of notions and questions.

In the end, an eclipse of sorrow
shrouded his sun as he peered
into darkness. Bewildered and
mute, he failed to grasp the
best of himself lived on in his
children and grandchildren,
redemption enough for his struggles.

# THE GARDEN AT AGE 70

What we've lost is counted
in daydreams, imagining
what might have been
or who we'd be if time
could roll back to innocence.

Perennials swagger, boasting
confidence and color each spring.
Optimism is everywhere.

But  we feel more annual now and
uneasy.  Flowers fade, shrinking
from haughty display.  Prior
certainties are brittle leaves,
wavering in the wind.

Fall heralds reluctant concessions.
Promises of upcoming germination
in another season linger fiercely.

## AT MEYERS' BAY

Pulling the door closed for the last time,
I shiver in a draft of grandfather's presence.
In days past, the front room was reserved
for reading Dickens and wondering if we'd
become the heroes of our own lives.

All seasons looked to the Bay for portents.
Windows arrayed under a green roof
gave seasonal perspective, witness
to gentle deeds and lost opportunities.
Promises of the possible were celebrated.

What remains now is what remains.
There are tales here, for children's children,
of sharing shelter from old storms.

# LEAVE-TAKING

Oak trees extend skeletal arms
across a somber sky as fall leaves
chuckle and crackle underfoot,
acquiescing to destiny.

Elephants, at the end, stagger
toward the shadows of ancestral
ground to gallantly disappear
from influence.

But there is no sanctuary for your
leave-taking. Dignity is forfeit
as pain, like the wind, comes
from nowhere and everywhere

to seek you out and scatter about
each ragged hope for a serene
departure.

# SEARCHING FOR SHED ANTLERS IN MARCH

*for Suzanne*

When the dull morning becomes sunshine
on snow, we head out in search of antlers
shed by deer too preoccupied to sense their loss.
Trails extend through trees, converging
at times before veering off over another hill.
Scat lends dark accent to furrows of snow
and crisscrosses patches of exposed ground
on south facing slopes.  Newly uncovered prairie
lies brittle and brown, exhausted by the winter.

We exclaim each time another antler is found,
eagerly counting points and our good fortune.
Someone asks how a deer, having lost its crown,
becomes whole again.  Much occurs behind our
backs.

Good things can follow loss, like insight and acceptance.
A new season unfolds.  Soon we'll seek pasque flowers
hidden among the hopeful grasses of spring.

**The following previously published poems in this collection are reprinted with permission:**

*The Garden at Age 70* -- JAMA, July 24, 2018

*The Trojans* -- in *Primary Care* (Bello & Coulehan, editors), University of Iowa Press, 2006

*On Depression* -- in *The Call to Care*, Ex Machina Publishing Company, 2006

*Searching for Shed Antlers in March* -- *South Dakota Magazine*, March/April 2005

*At Meyers Bay* -- in *Voices of Pogemama* (Ann Ryan), 2005

*Dementia Undone* -- in *Starting from Here*, Ex Machina Publishing Company, 1996

# Acknowledgements
## & APPRECIATION

CARL GRUPP: visual art

*The Road to Chamberlain* (page 2)
*Gimme a Vowel* (page 14)
*Eye before E except after Sea* (page26)
*Knight Death + My Devils* (page 36)
*No Pentamenti* (page 48)

MARIANNE LARSEN: photography

MARY SELVIG: art prep and framing

JASON FREEMAN: editing and conceptual design

CHRIS TAYLOR: creative design

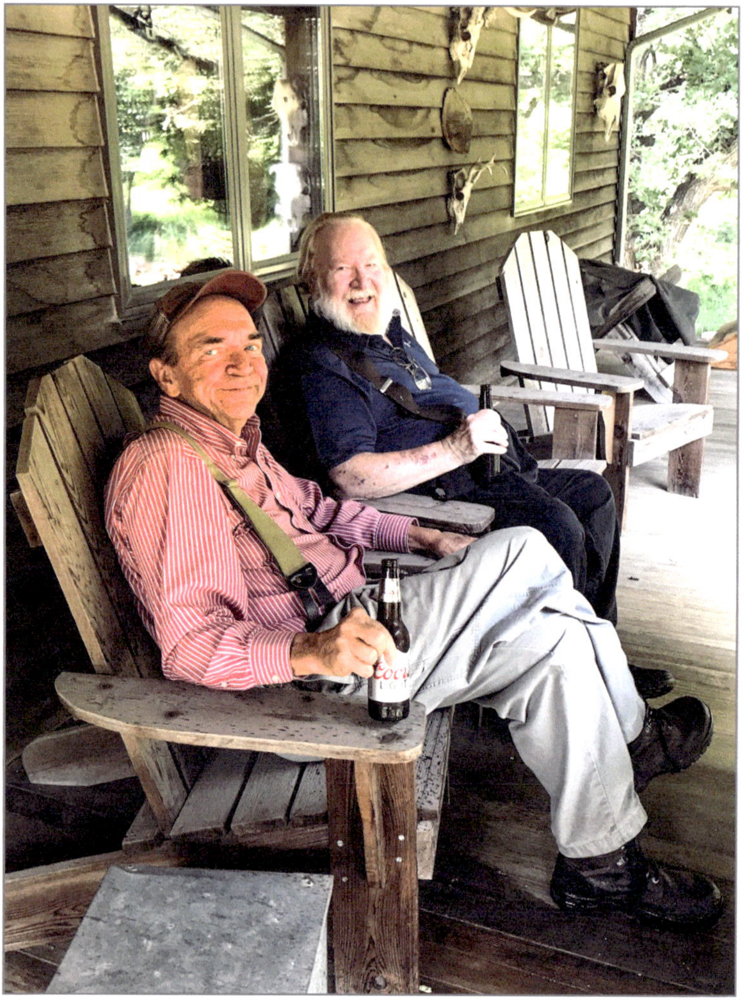

## ABOUT THE AUTHOR

Jerome W. Freeman is a practicing neurologist and educator. He is on the faculty of Sanford USD School of Medicine and an adjunct faculty of Augustana University. He has a particular interest in biomedical ethics and in the use of literature for teaching about illness, patients and clinicians. His previous publications include three books of poetry: Something at Last (1993), Easing the Edges (1994) and Starting from Here (1996); three books of essays: Come and See (1995), Colors of Care (2005) and Bringing Kindness to Medicine (2014); and sections of an anthology, The Call to Care (1999).

## ABOUT THE ARTIST

Carl Grupp is a preeminent artist and educator. He was a professor of art at Augustana University for 35 years and served as a mentor for many students. His work has included lithography and painting, and he has donated over 350 images to the Eide-Dalrymple Gallery at Augustana. Carl has wide-ranging interests including literature and jazz. He is a great friend to many people in the Sioux Falls region and across the country.

# *Praise For*

## THE COLORS OF CARE
## BY DR. FREEMAN

"This collection is a delight to read. Dr. Freeman has mastered the art of the short personal essay in which he writes about a single observation or incident that sheds light on an aspect of the human condition. In these essays Dr. Freeman employs his medical sensibility to imbue new meaning to a '58 Ford pickup, his father-in-law's garden, Andrew Wyeth's paintings, and an idiosyncratic bolo tie. He also reflects on patients and the foibles of medical practitioners. In every case his gentle wit and clear writing welcome the reader. And if the reader is anything like me, he or she immediately wants to join this master storyteller, as if they were sitting together on the front porch, and listen. I don't know whether the layperson will learn what 'those doctors' are thinking', but he or she will certainly learn--and be charmed and enlightened by--what this doctor is thinking."

**JACK COULEHAN, MD**
Author of *Medicine Stone*
Editor of *Chekhov's Doctors*

"This might be the most edifying book you'll read this year. Through short reflections on his experience, Dr. Freeman brings one face to face with the human aspects of medicine. I highly recommend this collection to physicians, patients, and anyone who will ever be either."

**MARK G. KUCZEWSKI, PhD**
Director, Neiswanger Institute for Bioethics
Stritch School of Medicine, Loyola University Chicago

Made in the USA
Monee, IL
05 November 2026

67383931R00043